MW00811213

The Fastest Pegan Diet Recipes for Beginners

Cookies, Cakes, Drinks –Sweety Pegan Recipes

Emy Fit

Table of Contents

Strawberry Ice Cream

Preparation Time: 5 minutes
Cooking Time: 5 minutes

Servings: 3

Ingredients:

- Stevia – ½ cup

- Lemon juice – 1 Tbsp.

- Non-dairy coffee creamer – ¾ cup

- Strawberries – 10 oz.

- Crushed ice – 1 cup

Directions:

1. Blend everything in a blender until smooth.

2. Freeze until frozen.
3. Serve.

Nutrition:

Calories: 94.4;

Fat: 6g;

Carb: 8.3g;

Phosphorus: 25mg;

Potassium: 108mg;

Sodium: 25mg;

Protein: 1.3g;

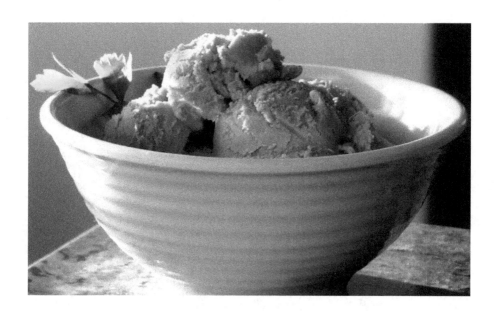

Cinnamon Custard

Preparation Time: 20 minutes

Cooking Time: 1 hour

Servings: 6

Ingredients:

- Unsalted butter, for greasing the ramekins

- Plain rice milk – 1 ½ cups

- Eggs – 4

- Granulated sugar – ¼ cup

- Pure vanilla extract – 1 tsp.

- Ground cinnamon – ½ tsp.

- Cinnamon sticks for garnish

Directions:

1. Preheat the oven to 325F.

2. Lightly grease six ramekins and place them in a baking dish. Set aside.
3. In a large bowl, whisk together the eggs, rice milk, sugar, vanilla, and cinnamon until the mixture is smooth.

4. Pour the mixture through a fine sieve into a pitcher.
5. Evenly divide the custard mixture among the ramekins.
6. Fill the baking dish with hot water until the water reaches halfway up the sides of the ramekins.
7. Bake for 1 hour or until the custards are set, and a knife inserted in the center comes out clean.
8. Remove the custards from the oven and take the ramekins out of the water.
9. Cool on the wire racks for 1 hour, then chill for 1 hour.
10. Garnish with cinnamon sticks and serve.

Nutrition:

Calories: 110;

Fat: 4g;
Carb: 14g;

Phosphorus: 100mg;

Potassium: 64mg;

Sodium: 71mg;

Protein: 4g;

Raspberry Brule

Preparation Time: 15 minutes

Cooking Time: 1 minute

Servings: 4

Ingredients:

- Light sour cream – ½ cup

- Plain cream cheese – ½ cup

- Brown sugar – ¼ cup, divided

- Ground cinnamon – ¼ tsp.

- Fresh raspberries – 1 cup

Directions:

1. Preheat the oven to broil.

2. In a bowl, beat together the cream cheese, sour cream, 2 tbsp. brown sugar and cinnamon for 4 minutes or until the mixture are very smooth and fluffy.
3. Evenly divide the raspberries among 4 (4-ounce) ramekins.
4. Spoon the cream cheese mixture over the berries and smooth the tops.
5. Sprinkle ½ tbsp. brown sugar evenly over each ramekin.

6. Place the ramekins on a baking sheet and broil 4 inches from the heating element until the sugar is caramelized and golden brown.
7. Cool and serve.

Nutrition:

Calories: 188;

Fat: 13g;

Carb: 16g;

Phosphorus: 60mg;

Potassium: 158mg;

Sodium: 132mg;

Tart Apple Granita

15 minutes, plus 4 hours freezing time
Cooking time: 0
Servings: 4
Ingredients:

- ½ cup granulated sugar

- ½ cup of water

- 2 cups unsweetened apple juice

- ¼ cup freshly squeezed lemon juice

Directions:

1. In a small saucepan over medium-high heat, heat the sugar and water.
2. Bring the mixture to a boil and then reduce the heat to low. Let it simmer for about 15 minutes or until the liquid has reduced by half.

3. Remove the pan from the heat and pour the liquid into a large shallow metal pan.

4. Let the liquid cool for about 30 minutes, and then stir in the apple juice and lemon juice.

5. Place the pan in the freezer.

6. After 1 hour, run a fork through the liquid to break up any ice crystals that have formed. Scrape down the sides as well.

7. Place the pan back in the freezer and repeat the stirring and scraping every 20 minutes, creating slush.

8. Serve when the mixture is completely frozen and looks like crushed ice, after about 3 hours.

Nutrition:

Calories: 157;

Fat: 0g;

Carbohydrates: 0g;

Phosphorus: 10mg;

Potassium: 141mg;

Sodium: 5mg;

Protein: 0g

Lemon-Lime Sherbet

Preparation Time:
5 minutes, plus 3 hours chilling time
Cooking time: 15 minutes
Ingredients:

- 2 cups of water

- 1 cup granulated sugar

- 3 tablespoons lemon zest, divided

- ½ cup freshly squeezed lemon juice

- Zest of 1 lime

- Juice of 1 lime

- ½ cup heavy (whipping) cream

Directions:

1. Place a large saucepan over medium-high heat and add the water, sugar, and two tablespoons of the lemon zest.

2. Bring the mixture to a boil and then reduce the heat and simmer for 15 minutes.

3. Transfer the mixture to a large bowl and add the remaining 1 tablespoon lemon zest, the lemon juice, lime zest, and lime juice.

4. Chill the mixture in the fridge until completely cold, about 3 hours.

5. Whisk in the heavy cream and transfer the mixture to an ice cream maker.

6. Freeze according to the manufacturer's instructions.

Nutrition:

Calories: 151;

Fat: 6g;

Carbohydrates: 26g;
Protein: 0g

Pavlova with Peaches

Preparation time: 30 minutes
Cooking time: 1 hour, plus cooling time
Servings: 3
Ingredients:

- 4 large egg whites, at room temperature
- ½ teaspoon cream of tartar
- 1 cup superfine sugar
- ½ teaspoon pure vanilla extract
- 2 cups drained canned peaches in juice

Directions:

1. Preheat the oven to 225°F.
2. Line a baking sheet with parchment paper; set aside.
3. In a large bowl, beat the egg whites for about 1 minute or until soft peaks form.
4. Beat in the cream of tartar.
5. Add the sugar, one tablespoon at a time, until the egg whites are very stiff and glossy. Do not overbeat.
6. Beat in the vanilla.
7. Evenly spoon the meringue onto the baking sheet so that you have eight rounds.
8. Use the back of the spoon to create an indentation in the middle of each round.
9. Bake the meringues for about 1 hour or until a light brown crust form.
10. Turn off the oven and let the meringues stand, still in the oven, overnight.
11. Remove the meringues from the sheet and place them on serving plates.

12. Spoon the peaches, dividing evenly into the centers of the meringues and serve.
13. Store any unused meringues in a sealed container at room temperature for up to 1 week.

Nutrition:
Calories: 132;
Fat: 0g;
Carbohydrates: 32g;
Protein: 2g

Tropical Vanilla Snow Cone

Preparation time: 15 minutes, plus freezing time
Cooking time: 0 minutes
Servings: 2
Ingredients:

- 1 cup pineapple
- 1 cup of frozen strawberries
- 6 tablespoons water
- 2 tablespoons granulated sugar
- 1 tablespoon vanilla extract

Directions:

1. In a large saucepan, mix together the peaches, pineapple, strawberries, water, and sugar over medium-high heat and bring to a boil.

2. Reduce the heat to low and simmer the mixture, occasionally stirring, for 15 minutes.

3. Remove from the heat and let the mixture cool completely, for about 1 hour.

4. Stir in the vanilla and transfer the fruit mixture to a food processor or blender.

5. Purée until smooth, and pour the purée into a 9-by-13-inch glass baking dish.

6. Cover and place the dish in the freezer overnight.

7. When the fruit mixture is completely frozen, use a fork to scrape the sorbet until you have flaked flavored ice.

8. Scoop the ice flakes into four serving dishes.

Nutrition:

Calories: 92;

Fat: 0g;

Carbohydrates: 22g;

Protein: 1g

Rhubarb Crumble

Preparation time: 15 minutes

Cooking time: 30 minutes

Servings: 6

Ingredients:

- Unsalted butter, for greasing the baking dish
- 1 cup all-purpose flour
- ½ cup brown sugar
- ½ teaspoon ground cinnamon
- ½ cup unsalted butter, at room temperature
- 1 cup chopped rhubarb
- 2 apples, peeled, cored, and sliced thin
- 2 tablespoons granulated sugar
- 2 tablespoons water

Directions:

1. Preheat the oven to 325°F.

2. Lightly grease an 8-by-8-inch baking dish with butter; set aside.

3. In a small bowl, stir together the flour, sugar, and cinnamon until well combined.

4. Add the butter and rub the mixture between your fingers until it resembles coarse crumbs.

5. In a medium saucepan, mix together the rhubarb, apple, sugar, and water over medium heat and cook for about 20 minutes or until the rhubarb is soft.

6. Spoon the fruit mixture into the baking dish and evenly top with the crumble.

7. Bake the crumble for 20 to 30 minutes or until golden brown.

8. Serve hot.

Nutrition:

Calories: 450;

Fat: 23g;

Carbohydrates: 60g;

Protein: 4g

Gingerbread Loaf

Preparation time: 20 minutes

Cooking time: 1 hour

Servings: 16

Ingredients:

- Unsalted butter, for greasing the baking dish
- 3 cups all-purpose flour
- ½ teaspoon Ener-G baking soda substitute
- 2 teaspoons ground cinnamon
- 1 teaspoon ground allspice
- ¾ cup granulated sugar
- 1¼ cups plain rice milk
- 1 large egg
- ¼ cup olive oil
- 2 tablespoons molasses
- 2 teaspoons grated fresh ginger
- Powdered sugar, for dusting

Directions:

1. Preheat the oven to 350°F.

2. Lightly grease a 9-by-13-inch baking dish with butter; set aside.

3. In a large bowl, sift together the flour, baking soda substitute, cinnamon, and allspice.

4. Stir the sugar into the flour mixture.

5. In medium bowl, whisk together the milk, egg, olive oil, molasses, and ginger until well blended.

6. Make a well in the center of the flour mixture and pour in the wet ingredients.

7. Mix until just combined, taking care not to overmix.

8. Pour the batter into the baking dish and bake for about 1 hour or until a wooden pick inserted in the middle comes out clean.

9. Serve warm with a dusting of powdered sugar.

Nutrition:

Calories: 232;

Fat: 5g;

Carbohydrates: 42g;

Protein: 4g

Elegant Lavender Cookies

Preparation time: 10 minutes
Cooking time: 15 minutes
Servings: Makes 24 cookies

Ingredients:

- 5 dried organic lavender flowers, the entire top of the flower ½ cup granulated sugar
- 1 cup unsalted butter, at room temperature
- 2 cups all-purpose flour
- 1 cup of rice flour

Directions:

1. Strip the tiny lavender flowers off the main stem carefully and place the flowers and granulated sugar into a food processor or blender. Pulse until the mixture is finely chopped.

2. In a medium bowl, cream together the butter and lavender sugar until it is very fluffy.

3. Mix the flours into the creamed mixture until the mixture resembles fine crumbs.

4. Gather the dough together into a ball and then roll it into a long log.

5. Wrap the cookie dough in plastic and refrigerate it for about 1 hour or until firm.

6. Preheat the oven to 375°F.

7. Slice the chilled dough into ¼-inch rounds and refrigerate it for 1 hour or until firm.

8. Bake the cookies for 15 to 18 minutes or until they are a very pale, golden brown.

9. Let the cookies cool.

10. Store the cookies at room temperature in a sealed container for up to 1 week.

Nutrition:

Calories: 153;

Fat: 9g;

Carbohydrates: 17g;

Phosphorus: 18mg;

Potassium: 17mg;

Sodium: 0mg;

Protein: 1g

Carob Angel Food Cake

Preparation time: 30 minutes
Cooking time: 30 minutes
Servings: 16

Ingredients:
- ¾ cup all-purpose flour
- ¼ cup carob flour
- 1½ cups sugar, divided
- 12 large egg whites, at room temperature
- 1½ teaspoons cream of tartar
- 2 teaspoons vanilla

Directions:

1. Preheat the oven to 375°F.

2. In a medium bowl, sift together the all-purpose flour, carob flour, and ¾ cup of the sugar; set aside.

3. Beat the egg whites and cream of tartar with a hand mixer for about 5 minutes or until soft peaks form.

4. Add the remaining ¾ cup sugar by the tablespoon to the egg whites until all the sugar is used up and stiff peaks form.

5. Fold in the flour mixture and vanilla.

6. Spoon the batter into an angel food cake pan.

7. Run a knife through the batter to remove any air pockets.

8. Bake the cake for about 30 minutes or until the top springs back when pressed lightly.

9. Invert the pan onto a wire rack to cool.

10. Run a knife around the rim of the cake pan and remove the cake from the pan.

Nutrition:

Calories: 113;

Fat: 0g;

Carbohydrates: 25g;

Phosphorus: 11mg;

Potassium: 108mg;

Sodium: 42mg;

Protein: 3g

Old-Fashioned Apple Kuchen

Preparation time: 25 minutes
Cook time: 1 hour
Servings: 16
Ingredients:

- Unsalted butter, for greasing the baking dish

- 1 cup unsalted butter, at room temperature

- 2 cups granulated sugar

- 2 eggs, beaten

- 2 teaspoons pure vanilla extract

- 2 cups all-purpose flour

- 1 teaspoon Ener-G baking soda substitute

- 2 teaspoons ground cinnamon

- ½ teaspoon ground nutmeg

- Pinch ground allspice
-
  2 large apples, peeled, cored, and diced (about 3 cups)

Directions:

1. Preheat the oven to 350°F.

2. Grease a 9-by-13-inch glass baking dish; set aside.

3. Cream together the butter and sugar with a hand mixer until light and fluffy, for about 3 minutes.

4. Add the eggs and vanilla and beat until combined, scraping down the sides of the bowl, about 1 minute.

5. In a small bowl, stir together the flour, baking soda substitute, cinnamon, nutmeg, and allspice.

6. Add the dry ingredients to the wet ingredients and stir to combine.

7. Stir in the apple and spoon the batter into the baking dish.

8. Bake for about 1 hour or until the cake is golden.

9. Cool the cake on a wire rack.

10. Serve warm or chilled.

Nutrition:

Calories: 368;

Fat: 16g;

Carbohydrates: 53g;

Phosphorus: 46mg;

Potassium: 68mg;

Sodium: 15mg;

Protein: 3g

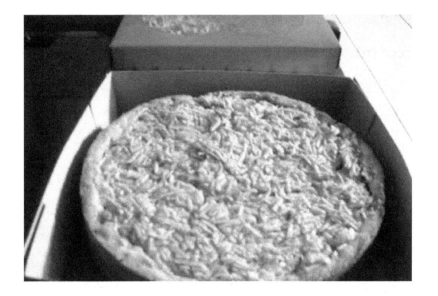

Dark Chocolate and Cherry Trail Mix

Preparation time: 5 minutes

Cooking time: 5 minutes

Servings: Makes 3 cups (¼ cup per serving)

Ingredients:

- 1 cup unsalted almonds

- 2/3 cup dried cherries

- ½ cup walnuts

- ½ cup sweet cinnamon-roasted chickpeas

- ¼ cup dark chocolate chips

Directions:

1. Combine the almonds, cherries, walnuts, chickpeas, and chocolate chips in an airtight container.

2. Store at room temperature for up to 1 week or in the freezer for up to 3 months.

Nutrition:

Calories: 174;

Total Fat: 12g;

Saturated Fat: 2g;

Cholesterol: 0mg;

Sodium: 18mg;

Carbohydrates: 16g;

Fiber: 4g;

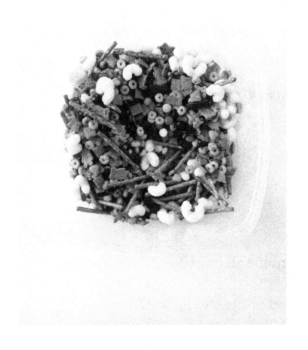

"Rugged" Coconut Balls

Preparation Time: 10minutes

Cooking time: 0minutes

Servings: 3

Ingredients:

- 1/3 cup coconut oil melted

- 1/3 cup coconut butter softened

- 2 oz. coconut, finely shredded, unsweetened

- 4 Tbsp. coconut palm sugar

- 1/2 cup shredded coconut

Directions:

1. Combine all ingredients in a blender.

2. Blend until soft and well combined.

3. Do a small ball roll in shredded coconut.

4. Place on a sheet lined with parchment paper and refrigerate overnight.

5. Keep coconut balls into sealed container in fridge up to one week.

Nutrition: Calories 226.89 Calories from Fat 190.39 | Total Fat 21.6g Saturated Fat 19.84g Cholesterol 0mg Sodium 17.19mg Potassium 45mg

Total Carbohydrates 9g Fiber 1.16g
Sugar 5.7g Protein 1g

Almond - Choco Cake

Preparation Time: 10minutes

Cooking time: 45minutes

Servings: 5

Ingredients:

- 1 1/2 cups of almond flour

- 1/3 cup almonds finely chopped

- 1/4 cup of cocoa powder unsweetened

- Pinch of salt

- 1/2 tsp. baking soda

- 2 Tbsp. almond milk

-
  1/2 cup Coconut oil melted
- 2 tsp. pure vanilla extract

- 1/3 cup brown sugar (packed)

Directions:

1. Preheat oven to 350 F.

2. Set the pan, and grease with a little melted coconut oil; set aside.

3. Stir the almond flour, chopped almonds, cocoa powder, salt, and baking soda in a bowl.

4. In a separate bowl, stir the remaining ingredients.

5. Merge the almond flour mixture with the almond milk mixture and stir well.

6. Place batter in a prepared cake pan.

7. Bake for 30 to 32 minutes...

8. Store the cake-slices a freezer, tightly wrapped in a double layer of plastic wrap and a layer of foil. It will keep on this way for up to a month.

Nutrition:

Calories 326.89

Calories from Fat 165.39 |

Total Fat 34.6g

Saturated Fat 29.84g

Cholesterol 0mg

Sodium 18.19mg

Potassium 45mg

Total Carbohydrates 9g

Fiber 1.16g

Sugar 5.7g

Protein 1g

Banana-Almond Cake

Preparation Time: 10minutes

Cooking time: 45minutes

Servings: 5

Ingredients

- 4 ripe bananas in chunks

- 3 Tbsps. honey or maple syrup

- 1 tsp. pure vanilla extract

- 1/2 cup almond milk

- 3/4 cup of self-rising flour

- 1 tsp. cinnamon

- 1 tsp. baking powder

- 1 pinch of salt

- 1/3 cup of almonds finely chopped

- Almond slices for decoration

Directions:
1. Preheat the oven to 400 F (air mode).

2. Oil a cake mold; set aside.

3. Add bananas into a bowl and mash with the fork.

4. Add honey, vanilla, almond, and stir well.

5. In a separate bowl, stir flour, cinnamon, baking powder, salt, the almonds broken, and mix with a spoon.

6. Transfer the mixture to prepared cake mold and sprinkle with sliced almonds.

7. Bake for 40-45 minutes.

8. Remove from the oven, and allow the cake to cool completely.

9. Cut cake into slices, place in tin foil, or an airtight container, and keep refrigerated up to one week.

Nutrition: Calories 326.89 Calories from Fat 145.39 | Total Fat 24.6g Saturated Fat 12.84g Cholesterol 0mg Sodium 20.19mg Potassium 32

Total Carbohydrates 9g Fiber 1.16g
Sugar 5.7g Protein 1g

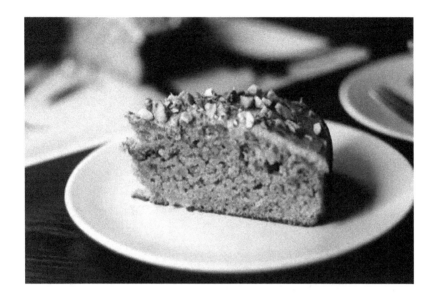

Banana-Coconut Ice Cream

Preparation Time: 15minutes

Cooking time: 0minutes

Servings: 5

Ingredients

- 1 cup coconut cream

- 1/2 cup Inverted sugar

- 2 large frozen bananas (chunks)

- 3 Tbsp. honey extracted

- 1/4 tsp. cinnamon powder

Directions:

1. Do the coconut cream with the inverted sugar in a bowl.

2. In a separate bowl, beat the banana with honey and cinnamon.

3. Incorporate the coconut whipped cream and banana mixture; stir well.

4. Cover the bowl and let cool in the refrigerator over the night.

5. Stir the mixture 3 to 4 times to avoid crystallization.

6. Keep frozen 1 to 2 months.

Nutrition:

Calories 126.89
Calories from Fat 245.39 |

Total Fat 34.6g

Saturated Fat 12.84g

Cholesterol 0mg

Sodium 20.19mg

Potassium 32

Total Carbohydrates 9g

Fiber 1.16g

Sugar 5.7g

Protein 1g

Coconut Butter Clouds Cookies

Preparation Time: 15minutes

Cooking time: 25minutes

Servings: 5

Ingredients

- 1/2 cup coconut butter softened

- 1/2 cup peanut butter softened

- 1/2 cup of granulated sugar

- 1/2 cup of brown sugar

- 2 Tbsp. chia seeds soaked in 4 tablespoons water

- 1/2 tsp. pure vanilla extract

- 1/2 tsp. baking soda

- 1/4 tsp. salt

- 1 cup of all-purpose flour

Directions:

1. Preheat oven to 360 F.

2. Add coconut butter, peanut butter, and both sugars in a mixing bowl.

3. Beat with a mixer until soft and sugar combined well.

4. Add soaked chia seeds and vanilla extract; beat.

5. Add baking soda, salt, and flour; beat until all ingredients are combined well.

6. With your hands, shape dough into cookies.

7. Arrange your cookies onto a baking sheet, and bake for about 10 minutes.

8. Remove cookies from the oven and allow cooling completely.

9. Sprinkle with icing sugar and enjoy your cookies.

10. Place cookies in an airtight container and keep refrigerated up to 10 days.

11. Nutrition:

Calories 226.89

Calories from Fat 255.39 |

Total Fat 34.6g

Saturated Fat 12.84g
Cholesterol 0mg

Sodium 10.19mg

Potassium 22

Total Carbohydrates 10g

Fiber 1.16g

Sugar 7.7g

Protein 5g

Choco Mint Hazelnut Bars

Preparation Time: 15minutes

Cooking time: 35minutes

Servings: 4

Ingredients

- 1/2 cup coconut oil, melted

- 4 Tbsp. cocoa powder

- 1/4 cup almond butter

- 3/4 cup brown sugar - (packed)

- 1 tsp. vanilla extract

- 1 tsp. pure peppermint extract

- Pinch of salt

- 1 cup shredded coconut

- 1 cup hazelnuts sliced

Directions:

1. Slice the hazelnuts in a food processor

2. Boil the and place it on low heat.

3. Put the coconut oil, cacao powder, almond butter, brown sugar, vanilla, peppermint extract, and salt in the top of a double boiler over hot (not boiling) water and constantly stir for 10 minutes.

4. Add hazelnuts and shredded coconut to the melted mixture and stir together.

5. Pour the mixture in a dish lined with parchment and freeze for several hours.

6. Remove from the freezer and cut into bars.

7. Store in airtight container or freezer bag in a freezer.

8. Let the bars at room temperature for 10 to 15 minutes before eating.

Nutrition:

Calories 126.89

Calories from Fat 155.39 |

Total Fat 34.6g

Saturated Fat 18.84g

Cholesterol 0mg

Sodium 15.19mg

Potassium 32

Total Carbohydrates 10g
Fiber 1.16g

Sugar 7.7g

Protein 5g

Coco-Cinnamon Balls

Preparation Time: 15minutes

Cooking time: 35minutes

Servings: 4

Ingredients

- 1 cup coconut butter softened

- 1 cup coconut milk canned

- 1 tsp. pure vanilla extract

- 3/4 tsp. cinnamon

- 1/2 tsp. nutmeg

- 2 Tbsp. coconut palm sugar (or granulated sugar)

- 1 cup coconut shreds

Directions:

1. Combine all ingredients (except the coconut shreds) in a heated bath - bain-marie.

2. Cook and stir until all ingredients are soft and well combined.

3. Remove bowl from heat, place into a bowl, and refrigerate until the mixture firmed up.

4. Form cold coconut mixture into balls, and roll each ball in the shredded coconut.

5. Store into a sealed container, and keep refrigerated up to one week.

Nutrition:

Calories 136.89

Fat 235.39 |

Total Fat 24.6g

Saturated Fat 19.84g

Cholesterol 0mg

Sodium 15.19mg

Potassium 32

Total Carbohydrates 10g

Fiber 2.16g

Sugar 7.7g

Protein 5g

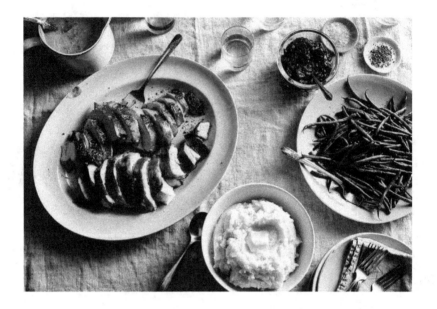

Express Coconut Flax Pudding

Preparation Time: 15minutes

Cooking time: 25minutes

Servings: 4

Ingredients

- 1 Tbsp. coconut oil softened

-
  1 Tbsp. coconut cream
- 2 cups coconut milk canned

- 3/4 cup ground flax seed

- 4 Tbsp. coconut palm sugar (or to taste)

Directions:

1. Press SAUTÉ button on your Instant Pot

2. Add coconut oil, coconut cream, coconut milk, and ground flaxseed.

3. Stir about 5 - 10 minutes.

4. Close lid into place and Start.

5. When the timer beeps, press "Cancel" and carefully flip the Quick Release valve to let the pressure out.

6. Add the palm sugar and stir well.

7. Taste and adjust sugar to taste.

8. Allow pudding to cool down completely.

9. Set the pudding in an airtight container and refrigerate for up to 2 weeks.

Nutrition:

Calories 126.89

Calories from Fat 124.39 |

Total Fat 14.6g

Saturated Fat 17.84g

Cholesterol 0mg

Sodium 18.19mg

Potassium 22

Total Carbohydrates 10g

Fiber 2.16g

Sugar 7.7g

Protein 5g

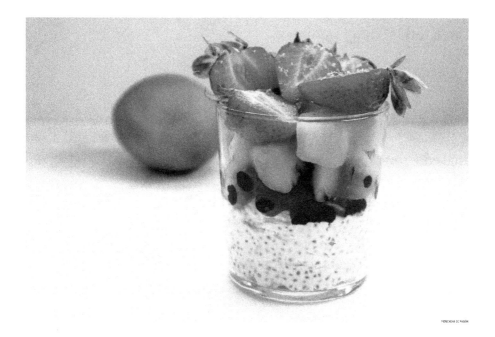

Full-Flavored Vanilla Ice Cream

Preparation Time: 15minutes

Cooking time: 0minutes

Servings: 4

Ingredients

- 1 1/2 cups canned coconut milk

- 1 cup coconut whipping cream

- 1 frozen banana cut into chunks

- 1 cup vanilla sugar

- 3 Tbsp. apple sauce

- 2 tsp. pure vanilla extract

- 1 tsp. Xanthan gum or agar-agar thickening agent

Directions:

1. Merge all ingredients; process until all ingredients combined well.

2. Place the ice cream mixture in a freezer-safe container with a lid over.
3. Freeze for at least 4 hours.

4. Remove frozen mixture to a bowl and beat with a mixer to break up the ice crystals.

5. Repeat this process 3 to 4 times.

6. Let the ice cream at room temperature for 15 minutes before serving.

Nutrition:

Calories 126.89

Calories from Fat 134.39 |

Total Fat 15.6g

Saturated Fat 19.84g

Cholesterol 0mg

Sodium 28.19mg

Potassium 22

Total Carbohydrates 10g

Fiber 2.16g

Sugar 7.7g

Protein 5g

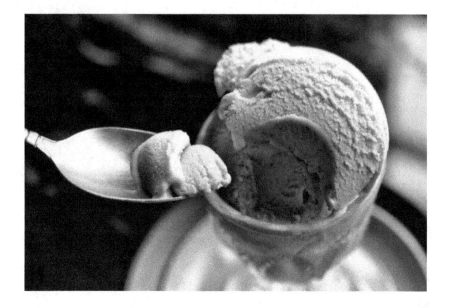

Irresistible Peanut Cookies

Preparation Time: 20minutes

Cooking time: 0minutes

Servings: 6

Ingredients

- 4 Tbsp. all-purpose flour

- 1 tsp. baking soda

- Pinch of salt

- 1/3 cup granulated sugar

- 1/3 cup peanut butter softened

- 3 Tbsp. applesauce

- 1/2 tsp. pure vanilla extract

Directions:

1. Preheat oven to 350 F.

2. Combine the flour, baking soda, salt, and sugar in a mixing bowl; stir.

3. Merge all remaining ingredients

4. Roll dough into cookie balls/patties.

5. Arrange your cookies onto greased (with oil or cooking spray) baking sheet.

6. Let cool before removing from tray.

7. Take out cookies from the tray and let cool completely.

8. Place your peanut butter cookies in an airtight container, and keep refrigerated up to 10 days.

Nutrition: Calories 116.89
Calories from Fat 114.39
Total Fat 18.6g

Saturated Fat 20.84g

Cholesterol 0mg

Sodium 12.19mg

Potassium 22

Total Carbohydrates 10g

Fiber 2.16g

Sugar 7.7g

Protein 5g

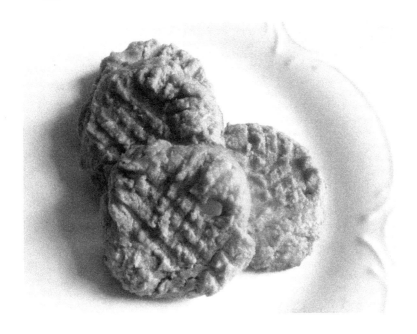

Murky Almond Cookies

Preparation Time: 10minutes

Cooking time: 15minutes

Servings: 6

Ingredients

- 4 Tbsp. cocoa powder

- 2 cups almond flour

- 1/4 tsp. salt

- 1/2 tsp. baking soda

- 5 Tbsp. coconut oil melted

- 2 Tbsp. almond milk

- 1 1/2 tsp. almond extract

- 1 tsp. vanilla extract

- 4 Tbsp. corn syrup or honey

Directions:

1. Preheat oven to 340 F degrees.

2. Grease a large baking sheet; set aside.

3. Merge the cocoa powder, almond flour, salt, and baking soda.

4. Merge the melted coconut oil, almond milk; almond and vanilla extract, and corn syrup or honey.

5. Merge the almond flour mixture with the almond milk mixture and stir well.

6. Roll tablespoons of the dough into balls, and arrange onto a prepared baking sheet.

7. Bake for 12 to 15 minutes.

8. Remove from the oven and transfer onto a plate lined with a paper towel.

9. Allow cookies to cool down completely and store in an airtight container at room temperature for about four days.

Nutrition:

Calories 16.89

Calories from Fat 19.39 |

Total Fat 18.6g

Saturated Fat 20.84g
Potassium 22

Total Carbohydrates 10g

Fiber 2.16g

Sugar 7.7g

Protein 5g

Orange Semolina Halva

Preparation Time: 10minutes

Cooking time: 25minutes

Servings: 6

Ingredients

- 6 cups fresh orange juice

- Zest from 3 oranges

- 3 cups brown sugar

- 1 1/4 cup semolina flour

- 1 Tbsp. almond butter (plain, unsalted)

- 4 Tbsp. ground almond

- 1/4 tsp. cinnamon

Directions:

1. Heat the orange juice, orange zest with brown sugar in a pot.

2. Let the sugar dissolved.

3. Add the semolina flour and cook over low heat for 15 minutes; stir occasionally.

4. Add almond butter, ground almonds, and cinnamon, and stir well.

5. Cook, frequently stirring, for further 5 minutes.

6. Transfer the halva mixture into a mold, let it cool and refrigerate for at least 4 hours.

7. Keep refrigerated in a sealed container for one week.

Nutrition:

Calories 16.89

Calories from Fat 19.39 |

Total Fat 18.6g

Saturated Fat 20.84g

Cholesterol 0mg

Sodium 12.19mg

Potassium 22

Total Carbohydrates 10g

Fiber 2.16g

Sugar 7.7g

Protein 5g

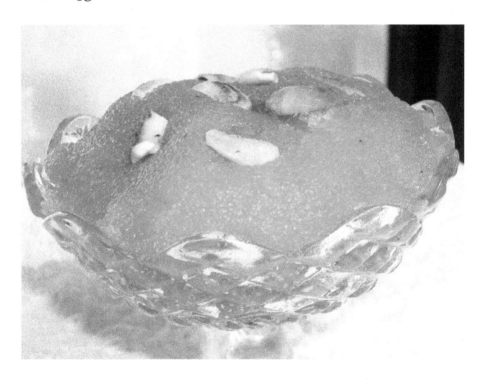

Seasoned Cinnamon Mango Popsicles

Preparation Time: 15minutes

Cooking time: 0minutes
Servings: 6

Ingredients

- 1 1/2 cups of mango pulp

- 1 mango cut in cubes

- 1 cup brown sugar (packed)

- 2 Tbsp. lemon juice freshly squeezed

- 1 tsp. cinnamon

- 1 pinch of salt

Directions:

1. Add all ingredients into your blender.

2. Blend until brown sugar dissolved.

3. Pour the mango mixture evenly in Popsicle molds or cups.

4. Insert sticks into each mold.

5. Place molds in a freezer, and freeze for at least 5 to6 hours.

6. Before serving, un-mold easy your popsicles placing molds under lukewarm water.

Nutrition: Calories 16.89 Calories from Fat 19.39 | Total Fat 18.6g Saturated Fat 20.84g Cholesterol 0mg Sodium 12.19mg Potassium 22

Total Carbohydrates 10g Fiber 2.16g
Sugar 7.7g Protein 5g

Strawberry Molasses Ice Cream

Preparation Time: 20minutes

Cooking time: 0minutes

Servings: 9

Ingredients

- 1 lb. strawberries

- 3/4 cup coconut palm sugar

- 1 cup coconut cream

- 1 Tbsp. molasses

- 1 tsp. balsamic vinegar

- 1/2 tsp. agar-agar

- 1/2 tsp. pure strawberry extract

Directions:
1. Add strawberries, date sugar, and the balsamic vinegar in a blender; blend until completely combined.

2. Place the mixture in the refrigerator for one hour.

3. In a mixing bowl, beat the coconut cream with an electric mixer to make a thick mixture.

4. Add molasses, balsamic vinegar, agar-agar, and beat for further one minute or until combined well.

5. Add the strawberry mixture and beat again for 2 minutes.

6. Pour ice cream mix into an ice cream maker, turn on the machine, and churn according to manufacturer's directions.

7. Keep frozen in a freezer-safe container (with plastic film and lid over).

Nutrition:

Calories 16.89

Calories from Fat 19.39 |

Total Fat 18.6g

Saturated Fat 20.84g

Cholesterol 0mg

Sodium 12.19mg

Potassium 22

Total Carbohydrates 10g

Fiber 2.16g

Sugar 7.7g

Protein 5g

Strawberry-Mint Sorbet

Preparation Time: 15minutes

Cooking time: 0minutes

Servings: 6

Ingredients

- 1 cup of granulated sugar

- 1 cup of orange juice

- 1 lb. frozen strawberries

- 1 tsp. pure peppermint extract

Directions:

1. Add sugar and orange juice in a saucepan.

2. Stir over high heat and boil for 5 minutes or until sugar dissolves.

3. Remove from the heat and let it cool down.

4. Add strawberries into a blender, and blend until smooth.

5. Pour syrup into strawberries, add peppermint extract and stir until all ingredients combined well.

6. Transfer mixture to a storage container, cover tightly, and freeze until ready to serve.

Nutrition:

Calories 16.89

Calories from Fat 1.39 |

Total Fat 12.6g
Saturated Fat 2.84g

Cholesterol 0mg

Sodium 1.19mg

Potassium 22

Total Carbohydrates 10g

Fiber 2.16g

Sugar 33g

Protein 5g

Vegan Choco - Hazelnut Spread

Preparation Time: 15minutes

Cooking time: 0minutes

Servings: 5

Ingredients

- 1 cup hazelnuts soaked

- 4 Tbsp. dry cacao powder

- 4 Tbsp. Maple syrup

- 1 tsp. pure vanilla extract

- 1/4 tsp. kosher salt

- 4 Tbsp. almond milk

Directions:

1. Soak hazelnuts with water overnight.

2. Add soaked hazelnuts along with all remaining ingredients in a food processor.

3. Process for about 10 minutes or until a cream gets the desired consistency.

4. Keep the spread in a sealed container refrigerated up to 2 weeks.

Nutrition:

Calories 16.89

Calories from Fat 4.39 |

Total Fat 6.6g

Saturated Fat 3.84g

Cholesterol 0mg

Sodium 5.19mg

Potassium 22

Total Carbohydrates 10g

Fiber 2.16g

Sugar 43g

Protein 5g

Vegan Exotic Chocolate Mousse

Preparation Time: 10minutes

Cooking time: 0minutes

Servings: 4
Ingredients:

- 2 frozen bananas chunks

- 2 avocados

- 1/3 cup of dates

- 4 Tbsp. cocoa powder

- 1/2 cup of fresh orange juice

- Zest, from 1 orange

Directions:

1. Add bananas, avocado, and dates in a food processor.

2. Process for about 2 to 3 minutes until combined well.

3. Add cocoa powder, orange juice, and orange zest; process for further one minute.

4. Place cream in a glass jar or container and keep refrigerated up to one week.

5. Nutrition: Facts

Nutrition:

Calories 16.89

Calories from Fat 4.39 |

Total Fat 5.6g

Saturated Fat 2.84g

Cholesterol 0mg

Sodium 7.19mg

Potassium 32

Total Carbohydrates 10g

Fiber 2.16g

Sugar 43g

Protein 5g

Vegan Lemon Pudding

Preparation Time: 20minutes

Cooking time: 0minutes

Servings: 6

Ingredients

- 2 cups almond milk

- 3 Tbsp. of corn flour

- 2 Tbsp. of all-purpose flour

- 1 cup of sugar granulated

- 1/4 cup almond butter (plain, unsalted)

- 1 tsp. lemon zest

- 1/3 cup fresh lemon juice

Directions:

1. Add the almond milk with corn flour, flour, and sugar in a saucepan.

2. Cook, frequently stirring, until sugar dissolved, and all ingredients combine well (for about 5 to 7 minutes over medium heat).

3. Add the almond butter, lemon zest, and lemon juice.

4. Cook, frequently stirring, for further 5 to 6 minutes.

5. Remove the lemon pudding from the heat and allow it to cool completely.

6. Pour into the sealed container and keep refrigerated up to one week.

Nutrition: Calories 16.89 Calories from Fat 7.39 | Total Fat 3.6g Saturated Fat 1.84g Cholesterol 0mg Sodium 7.19mg Potassium432

Total Carbohydrates 20g Fiber 1.16g
Sugar 24g Protein 5g

Vitamin Blast Tropical Sherbet

Preparation Time: 15minutes

Cooking time: ominutes

Servings: 8

Ingredients

- 4 cups mangos pitted and cut into 1/2-inch dice

- 1 papaya cut into 1/2-inch dice

- 1/4 cup granulated sugar or honey (optional)

- 1 cup pineapple juice canned

- 1/4 cup coconut milk

- 2 Tbsp. coconut cream

- 1 fresh lime juice

Directions:

1. Add all ingredients into your food processor; process until all ingredients smooth and combine well.

2. Put the mixture to a bowl, and cover

3. Remove the sherbet mixture from the fridge, stir well, and pour in a freezer-safe container (with plastic film and lid over).

4. Keep frozen.

5. Let the sherbet at room temperature for 15 minutes before serving.

Nutrition:

Calories 16.89

Calories from Fat 9.39 |

Total Fat 2.6g
Saturated Fat 3.84g

Cholesterol 0mg

Sodium 7.15mg

Potassium132

Total Carbohydrates 15g

Fiber 1.16g

Sugar 24g

Protein 5g

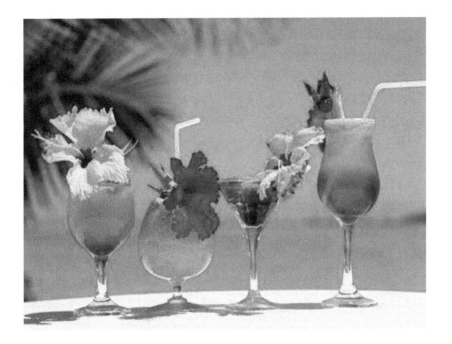

Walnut Vanilla Popsicles

Preparation Time: 15minutes

Cooking time: 0minutes

Servings: 7

Ingredients

- 1 1/2 cup finely sliced walnuts

- 4 cups of almond milk

- 4 Tbsp. brown sugar (packed)

- 1 scoop protein powder (pea or soy)

- 2 tsp. pure vanilla extract

Directions:

1. Add all ingredients in your high-speed blender and blend until smooth and combined well.

2. Pour the mixture in Popsicle molds and insert the wooden stick into the middle of each mold.

3. Freeze until your ice popsicles are completely frozen.

4. Serve and enjoy!

Nutrition:

Calories 16.89

Calories from Fat 9.39 |

Total Fat 2.6g

Saturated Fat 3.84g

Cholesterol 0mg

Sodium 7.15mg

Potassium122

Total Carbohydrates 15g

Fiber 1.16g

Sugar 34g

Protein 5g

Carrot-Ginger Soup

Preparation Time: 5minutes

Cooking time: 60minutes

Servings: 5

Ingredients:

- 2 (10-ounce) packages frozen carrots

- 2 cans diced tomatoes

- 1 medium yellow onion, diced

- 1-piece fresh ginger

- 1.1/2 teaspoons minced garlic (3 cloves)

- Zest and juice of 1 lemon

- 2 vegetable bouillon cubes

- 3.1/2 cups water

- 2 tablespoons vegan sour cream

- Pinch salt

- Freshly ground black pepper

Directions:

1. Combine the carrots, diced tomatoes, onion, ginger, garlic, lemon zest and juice, bouillon cubes, and water in a slow cooker; mix well

2. Shut down and cook on low heat.

3. Purée using an immersion blender (or with a regular blender, working in batches).

4. Stir in the vegan sour cream and season with salt and pepper.

Nutrition:

Calories: 137

Total fat: 6g

Saturated fat: 9g

Sodium: 138mg

Carbs: 18g

Fiber: 8g

Protein: 6g

Blueberry Cake

Preparation Time: 10 Minutes

Cooking Time: 30 Minutes

Servings: 6

Ingredients:

- 2 cups almond flour
- 3 cups blueberries
- 1 cup walnuts, chopped
- 3 tablespoons stevia
- 1 teaspoon vanilla extract
- 2 eggs, whisked
- 2 tablespoons avocado oil
- 1 teaspoon baking powder
- Cooking spray

Directions:

1. In a bowl, blend the flour plus the blueberries, walnuts and the other ingredients except for the cooking spray, and stir well.

2. Grease a cake pan with the cooking spray, pour the cake mix inside, introduce everything in the oven at 350 degrees F and bake for 30 minutes.
3. Cool the cake down, slice and serve.

Nutrition:

Calories 225

Fat 9

Fiber 4.5

Carbs 10.2

Protein 4.5

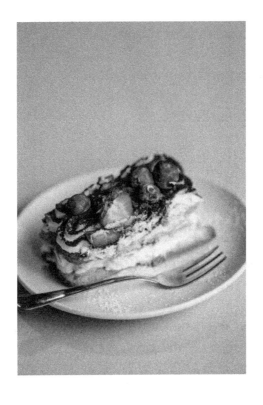

Almond Peaches Mix

Preparation Time: 10 Minutes

Cooking Time: 10 Minutes

Servings: 4

Ingredients:

- 1/3 cup almonds, toasted
- 1/3 cup pistachios, toasted
- 1 teaspoon mint, chopped
- ½ cup of coconut water
- 1 teaspoon lemon zest, grated
- 4 peaches, halved
- 2 tablespoons stevia

Directions:

1. In a pan, combine the peaches with the stevia and the rest of the ingredients.
2. Simmer over medium heat for 10 minutes.
3. Divide into bowls and serve cold.

Nutrition:

Calories 135

Fat 4.1

Fiber 3.8

Carbs 4.1

Protein 2.3

Spiced Peaches

Preparation Time: 5 minutes

Cooking Time: 10 minutes

Servings: 2

Ingredients:

- Canned peaches with juices – 1 cup

- Cornstarch – ½ tsp.

- Ground cloves – 1 tsp.

- Ground cinnamon – 1 tsp.

- Ground nutmeg – 1 tsp.

- Zest of ½ lemon

- Water – ½ cup

Directions:

1. Drain peaches.

2. Combine cinnamon, cornstarch, nutmeg, ground cloves, and lemon zest in a pan on the stove.

3. Heat on medium heat and add peaches.
4. Bring to a boil, decrease the heat then simmer for 10 minutes.
5. Serve.

Nutrition:

Calories: 70;

Fat: 0g;

Carb: 14g;
Phosphorus: 23mg;

Potassium: 176mg;

Sodium: 3mg;

Protein: 1g

Pumpkin Cheesecake Bar

Preparation Time: 10 minutes

Cooking Time: 50 minutes

Servings: 4

Ingredients:

- Unsalted butter – 2 ½ Tbsps.

- Cream cheese – 4 oz.

- All-purpose white flour – ½ cup

- Golden brown sugar – 3 Tbsps.

- Granulated sugar – ¼ cup

- Pureed pumpkin – ½ cup

- Egg whites - 2

- Ground cinnamon – 1 tsp.

- Ground nutmeg – 1 tsp.

- Vanilla extract – 1 tsp.

Directions:

1. Preheat the oven to 350F.

2. Mix brown sugar and flour in a container.
3. Mix in the butter to form 'breadcrumbs.'
4. Place ¾ of this mixture in a dish.
5. Bake in the oven for 15 minutes. Remove and cool.
6. Lightly whisk the egg and fold in the cream cheese, sugar, pumpkin, cinnamon, nutmeg, and vanilla until smooth.
7. Pour this mixture over the oven-baked base and sprinkle with the rest of the breadcrumbs from earlier.

8. Bake for 30 to 35 minutes more.
9. Cool, slice, and serve.

Nutrition:

Calories: 248;

Fat: 13g;

Carb: 33g;

Phosphorus: 67mg;

Potassium: 96mg;

Sodium: 146mg;

Protein: 4g

Blueberry Mini Muffins

Preparation Time: 10 minutes

Cooking Time: 35 minutes

Servings: 4

Ingredients:

- Egg whites – 3

-
  All-purpose white flour – ¼ cup
- Coconut flour – 1 Tbsp.

- Baking soda – 1 tsp.

- Nutmeg – 1 Tbsp. grated

- Vanilla extract – 1 tsp.

- Stevia – 1 tsp.

- Fresh blueberries – ¼ cup

Directions:

1. Preheat the oven to 325F.

2. Mix all the ingredients in a bowl.

3. Divide the batter into four and spoon into a lightly oiled muffin tin.

4. Bake in the oven for 15 to 20 minutes or until cooked through.
5. Cool and serve.

Nutrition:

Calories: 62;

Fat: 0g;

Carb: 9g;

Phosphorus: 103mg;

Potassium: 65mg;

Sodium: 62mg;

Protein: 4g;

Vanilla Custard

Preparation Time: 7 minutes

Cooking Time: 10 minutes

Servings: 10

Ingredients:

- Egg – 1

- Vanilla – 1/8 tsp.

- Nutmeg – 1/8 tsp.

- Almond milk – ½ cup

- Stevia - 2 Tbsp.

Directions:

1. Scald the milk, then let it cool a little.

2. Break the egg into a bowl and beat it with the nutmeg.
3. Add the scalded milk, the vanilla, and the sweetener to taste. Mix well.

4. Place the bowl in a baking pan filled with ½ deep of water.
5. Bake for 30 minutes at 325F.
6. Serve.

Nutrition:

Calories: 167.3;

Fat: 9g;

Carb: 11g;

Phosphorus: 205mg;

Potassium: 249mg;

Sodium: 124mg;
Protein: 10g;

Chocolate Chip Cookies

Preparation Time: 7 minutes

Cooking Time: 10 minutes

Servings: 10

Ingredients:

- Semi-sweet chocolate chips – ½ cup

- Baking soda – ½ tsp.

- Vanilla – ½ tsp.

- Egg – 1

- Flour – 1 cup

- Margarine – ½ cup

- Stevia – 4 tsp.

Directions:

1. Sift the dry ingredients.

2. Cream the margarine, stevia, vanilla, and egg with a whisk.
3. Add flour mixture and beat well.
4. Stir in the chocolate chips, then drop a teaspoonful of the mixture over a greased baking sheet.

5. Bake the cookies for about 10 minutes at 375F.
6. Cool and serve.

Nutrition:

Calories: 106.2;

Fat: 7g;

Carb: 8.9g;

Phosphorus: 19mg;

Potassium: 28mg;

Sodium: 98mg;

Protein: 1.5g;

Baked Peaches with Cream Cheese

Preparation Time: 10 minutes

Cooking Time: 15 minutes

Servings: 4

Ingredients:

- Plain cream cheese – 1 cup

- Crushed meringue cookies – ½ cup

- Ground cinnamon – ¼ tsp.

- Pinch ground nutmeg

- Canned peach halves – 8, in juice

- Honey – 2 Tbsp.

Directions:

1. Preheat the oven to 350F.

2. Line a baking sheet with parchment paper. Set aside.

3. In a small bowl, stir together the meringue cookies, cream cheese, cinnamon, and nutmeg.

4. Spoon the cream cheese mixture evenly into the cavities in the peach halves.
5. Place the peaches on the baking sheet and bake for 15 minutes or until the fruit is soft and the cheese is melted.
6. Remove the peaches from the baking sheet onto plates.
7. Drizzle with honey and serve.

Nutrition:

Calories: 260;

Fat: 20;

Carb: 19g;

Phosphorus: 74mg;

Potassium: 198mg;

Sodium: 216mg;

Protein: 4g;

Bread Pudding

Preparation Time: 15 minutes

Cooking Time: 40 minutes

Servings: 6

Ingredients:

- Unsalted butter, for greasing the baking dish

- Plain rice milk – 1 ½ cups

- Eggs – 2

- Egg whites – 2

- Honey – ¼ cup

- Pure vanilla extract – 1 tsp.

- Cubed white bread – 6 cups

Directions:

1. Grease an 8-by-8-inch baking dish with butter. Set it aside.

2. In a bowl, whisk together the eggs, egg whites, rice milk, honey, and vanilla.
3. Add the bread cubes and stir until the bread is coated.

4. Transfer the mixture to the baking dish and cover with plastic wrap.
5. Store the dish in the refrigerator for at least 3 hours.
6. Preheat the oven to 325F.
7. Take away the plastic wrap from the baking dish, bake the pudding for 35 to 40 minutes, or golden brown.

8. Serve.

Nutrition:

Calories: 167;

Fat: 3g;

Carb: 30g;

Phosphorus: 95mg;

Potassium: 93mg;

Sodium: 189mg;

Protein: 6g;

Avocado, Spinach and Kale Soup

Preparation time: 10 minutes

Cooking time: 0 minutes

Servings: 4

Ingredients:

- 2 avocados, pitted, peeled and cut in halves

- 4 cups vegetable stock

- 2 tablespoons cilantro, chopped

- Juice of 1 lime

- 1 teaspoon rosemary, dried

- 1/2 cup spinach leaves

- 1/2 cup kale, torn

- Salt and black pepper to the taste

Directions

1. In a blender, combine the avocados with the stock and the other ingredients, pulse well, divide into bowls and serve for lunch.

Nutrition:

Calories: 124

Total fat: 9g

Saturated fat: 6g

Sodium: 158mg

Carbs: 18g

Fiber: 8g

Protein: 6g

Spinach and Broccoli Soup

Preparation time: 10 minutes

Cooking time: 20 minutes

Servings: 4

Ingredients:

- 3 shallots, chopped

- 1 tablespoon olive oil

- 2 garlic cloves, minced

- 1/2-pound broccoli florets

- 1/2-pound baby spinach

- Salt and black pepper to the taste

- 4 cups veggie stock

- 1 teaspoon turmeric powder

- 1 tablespoon lime juice

Directions:

2. Heat up a pot with the oil over medium high heat; add the shallots and the garlic and sauté for 5 minutes.

3. Add the broccoli, spinach and the other ingredients toss bring to a simmer and cook over medium heat for 15 minutes.

4. Ladle into soup bowls and serve.

Nutrition:

Calories: 124

Total fat: 9g

Saturated fat: 6g

Sodium: 158mg

Carbs: 18g

Fiber: 8g

Protein: 6g

Zucchini and Cauliflower Soup

Preparation time: 10 minutes

Cooking time: 25 minutes

Servings: 4

Ingredients:

- 4 scallions, chopped

- 1 teaspoon ginger, grated

- 2 tablespoons olive oil

- 1-pound zucchinis, sliced

- 2 cups cauliflower florets

- Salt and black pepper to the taste

- 6 cups veggie stock

- 1 garlic clove, minced

- 1 tablespoon lemon juice

- 1 cup coconut cream

Directions:

1. Heat up a pot with the oil over medium heat; add the scallions, ginger and the garlic and sauté for 5 minutes.

2. Add the rest of the ingredients, bring to a simmer and cook over medium heat for 20 minutes.

3. Blend everything using an immersion blender, ladle into soup bowls and serve.

Nutrition:

Calories: 114

Total fat: 8g

Saturated fat: 6g

Sodium: 128mg

Carbs: 18g

Fiber: 8g
Protein: 6g

CPSIA information can be obtained
at www.ICGtesting.com
Printed in the USA
BVHW090831240521
607631BV00013B/319

9 781802 694642